How to Get Rid Of Stretch Marks Naturally

Table of Contents

INTRODUCTION

Stretch marks appear when the skin is stretched and the collagen is weakened. This mostly occurs when the normal production circle of collagen is damaged or interrupted. The line-scars under the top layer of the skin referred to as stretch marks go through some stages of development: it starts with a red or pink mark on the skin; on the second stage a silvery line appears, often thin, and this might not be completely visible to the eye. The third brings about the bold stretch mark.

In most cases, stretch marks appear on the skin as a result of drastic weight gain or loss. They are found around the upper arms, buttocks, breasts, thighs and the abdominal wall. These lines have the tendency of covering large area of the body.

The main cause of stretch marks in women is pregnancy but other factors such as stress, heredity, drastic change in physical condition, use of new skin cream and obviously rapid growth are among the common causes of stretch marks.

CHAPTER ONE: Causes of Stretch Mark

The epidermis, dermis and hypodermis are the three main skin layers. Firstly, stretch marks form in the middle layer (dermis) as a result of stretched connective tissue—when this tissue gets stretched beyond its elastic limit due to continues contraction and expansion of the skin.

Stretched marks can also be caused by the increase in cortisone in the system. Cortisone, which is produced by the adrenal gland naturally, tends to reduce the skin's elasticity by making it loose. The circumstances common to developing stretch marks include:

Corticosteroid Creams

Some creams decrease the ability of the skin to stretch, therefore causing break when the skin is faced with strain. Naturally, the skin has a certain resistance to strain and forceful stretching, but the application of these creams reduces this flexibility. The Corticosteroid creams come first followed by the pills and lotions.

Adrenal Gland Disorders

Adrenal gland disorders reduce the amount of cortisone in the body, therefore causing stretch marks. Examples of these disorders include the Ehlers-Danlos syndrome, Marfan syndrome and the Cushing's syndrome.

Weight loss or gain

The effect of rapid weight gain or loss in developing stretch marks on the skin is common among teenagers. This happens among both genders and can be controlled easily.

Pregnancy

During pregnancy, there is a continual tugging and stretching when the baby is developing. Also, the body undergoes different phases of change which may result to weight gain and stress. These factors increase the tendency for women to develop stretch marks.

What increases your risk for developing stretch marks?

You are in greater risk for developing stretch marks;

When you become pregnant

When you have a history of delivering twins or large babies

When you are a woman

When you are overweight

When you use corticosteroid medications

When you have a family history of stretch marks

When you have regular or rapid weight loss or gain

When you have pale skin (example, being a Caucasian)

CHAPTER TWO: Medical Treatment Options

This is book is about the natural ways to get rid of stretch marks but before we get into that, let's look at the medical treatment options available:

Pulsed Dye Laser Therapy

This therapy is often used on newer formed stretched marks and the aim is to encourage the growth of elastin and collagen. Skin discoloration might occur when used on darker skins.

Microdermabrasion

This procedure is aimed at improving the appearance of the skin, and can be applied for older stretch marks. The skin is being polished with tiny crystals in order to reveal new skin, which should be more elastic than the older one with stretch marks.

Fractional Photothermolysis

Just like the pulsed dye laser therapy, fractional Photothermolysis also involves the use of laser. In this case, smaller parts of the skin are being targeted and cause less skin damage compared to the pulsed dye laser therapy.

The Excimer Laser

This is used to stimulate melanin (skin color) production in order to make the stretch mark match the color of the skin.

Tretinoin Cream

This includes Renova, Retin-A, etc., and this cream is used on new stretch marks. It helps give the skin elasticity by restoring the collagen. The process of restoring this fibrous protein using the Tretinoin cream may cause skin irritation, so pregnant women are advised to stay away from the use.

These prescriptions and procedures are mostly expensive and are not necessarily guaranteed to cure your stretch marks. There are so many natural methods you can use to get rid of stretch marks and also achieve a better skin color.

CHAPTER THREE: Natural Methods

Use of Lemon Juice

The natural acidic content of lemon juice helps reduce and heal not only stretch marks but acne scars. All you need is a fresh slice of lemon fruit.

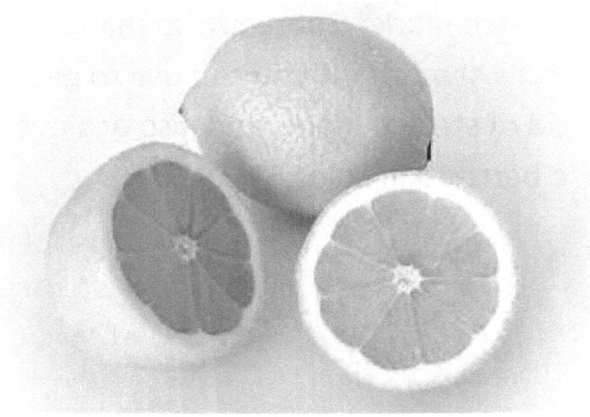

Procedure:

Step 1: Slice a moderately ripe lemon fruit into two.

Step 2: Using circular motions, rub one slice of the lemon onto the stretch marks, while pressing firmly to squeeze out the juice.

The procedure should take not more than ten minutes. Allow the juice to stay on the skin for another ten minutes before rinsing off with warm water.

Alternatively, extract fresh lemon juice and mix with the same quantity of cucumber juice, mix and apply the mixture. This is recommended for people with softer or sensitive skin.

Use of Potato Juice

Potato juice works in restoring and fostering growth of the skin cells due to its mineral and vitamin contents.

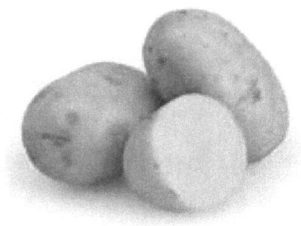

Procedure:

Step 1: Into thick slices, cut a medium-sized potato.

Step 2: Rub one of the potato slices on the stretch marks gently for 3 minutes. Use a moderate pressure to make sure the starch of the potato rubs deeply along the affected area of the skin.

Also, you can allow it for 10 minutes or so to dry off before washing with warm water.

Castor Oil

Apart from stretch marks, castor oil can be used to treat quite a number of skin problems including moles, pimples, age spots, dark spots, fine lines and wrinkles. The procedure used in getting rid of stretch marks is quiet simple and it works effectively.

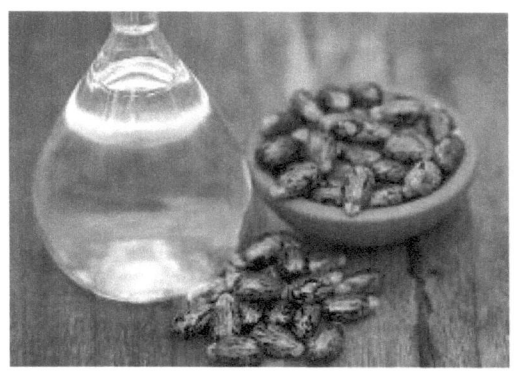

Procedure:

Step 1: Apply thick castor oil on the area affected and massage gently. The massage is best effective when done in circular motion, and it should last for 10 minutes minimum.

Step 2: Wrap the skin with cotton clothing, the thinner the better.

Step 3: Use a heating pad or a bottle of warm-hot water to apply heat to the skin. This should also last for 30 minutes, at least.

The same process should be repeated daily for the minimum of 3 weeks to experience significant result.

Sugar

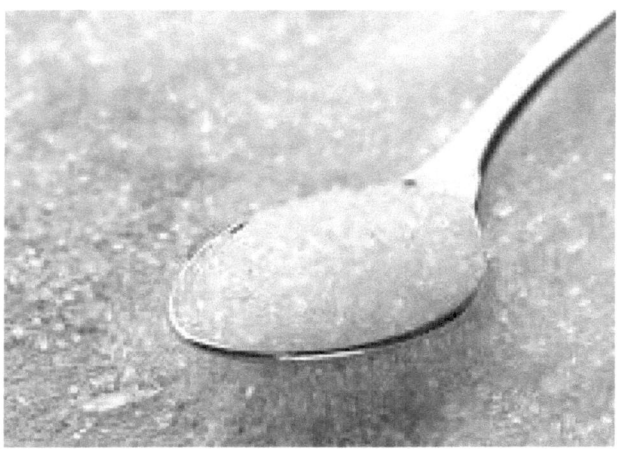

Step 1: Obtain one tablespoon of raw sugar and mix with almond oil. Add a few drops of lemon juice and mix. The mixture can be applied immediately to the affected skin and other skin areas.

Step 2: The procedure should be carried out once a day, few minutes before you take a shower. The mixture should stay on the skin for 5 to 10 minutes before you wash it off.

The longer and more consistent this procedure is being practiced, the better result to be obtained.

Egg whites

As a rich source of protein and amino acids, the egg whites alone can be used effectively to get rid of stretch marks.

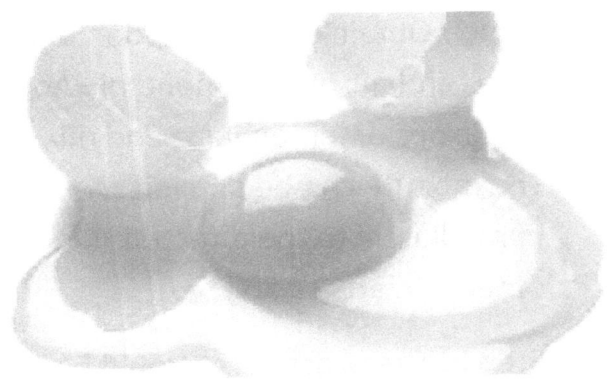

Procedures:

Step 1: Break two eggs and use a fork to whip the whites.

Step 2: Use water to clean the area of skin affected by stretch marks. Use a makeup brush to apply thick layer of egg whites.

Step 3: Allow for a while to dry up.

Use cold water to rinse the skin.

Step 4: You can apply olive oil immediately to keep the skin moisturized and toned.

The procedure should be repeated daily for two weeks for significant result.

CHAPTER FOUR: Home Remedies for Stretch Marks

Aloe Vera

Aloe Vera also has a soothing and healing properties and it is effective in treating several skin ailments.

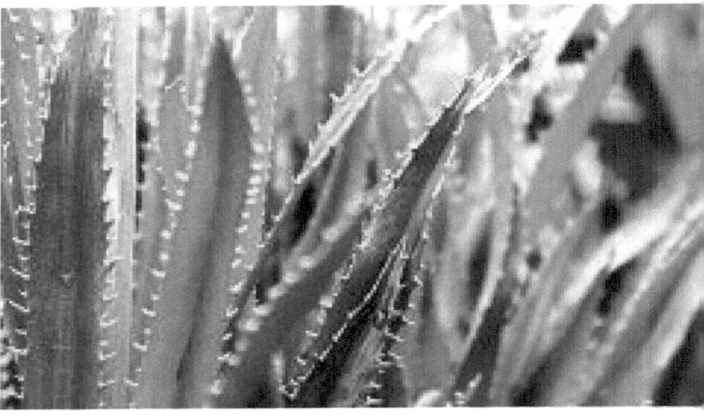

Method 1:

Rub Aloe Vera gel directly on the area affected by stretch marks, let it stay for 10 to 15 minutes and rinse with warm water.

Method 2:

Using this method you will need Aloe Vera gel (one-fourth cup), oil from 5 vitamin A capsules and oil from ten vitamin E capsules.

Mix the 3 substances together and rub continuously on the affected skin until you are sure it is absorbed.

Repeat once, daily or every other day.

Cocoa Butter

Cocoa butter is a natural moisturizer. It best works in nourishing the skin and helps in making the stretch marks fade.

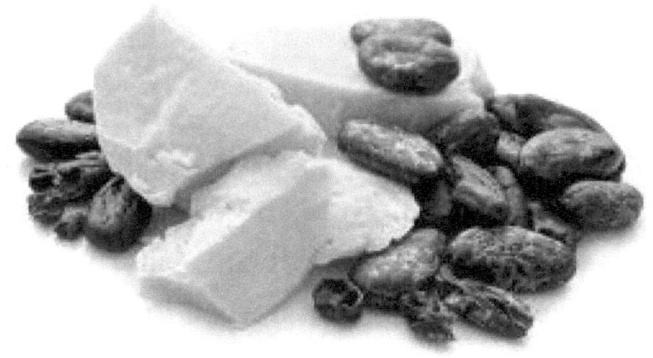

Method 1:

Simply apply the cocoa butter on the stretch marks two times a day.

This can be repeated for 3 weeks or more.

Method 2:

Get one tablespoon of vitamin E oil, another tablespoon of apricot kernel oil, 2 tablespoons of grated beeswax, one teaspoon of wheat germ oil and a half cup of cocoa butter.

Mix them together and heat until the grated beeswax melts. Apply to affected area 2 to 3 times daily.

It can be stored in the refrigerator in an airtight container.

Hydration and smoothness of the skin is assured when this mixture is used regularly.

Alfalfa Leaves

These leaves contain the complete eight essential amino acids required for a healthy skin. Also, nourishment of the skin is achieved due to the rich vitamin E and K, and protein.

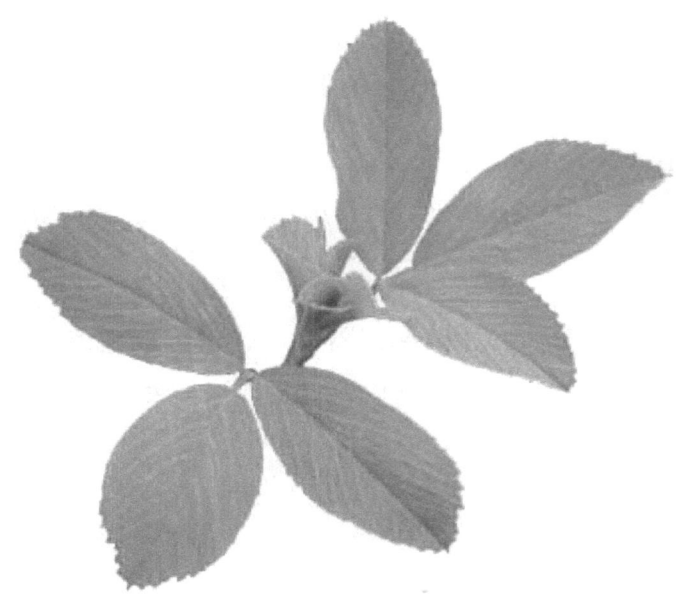

Procedure:

Step 1: Make an alfalfa paste by mixing alfalfa powder with chamomile oil. Obtain the powder first, put in a container and put a few drops of chamomile oil to make a paste.

Step 2: Rub the mixture on the skin area affected and massage; to be repeated 3 times daily.

Also, repeating daily for 2 weeks or more will give better results.

Olive oil

Olive oil has antioxidants and high nutrient content. It can be used for miniaturization and skin exfoliation.

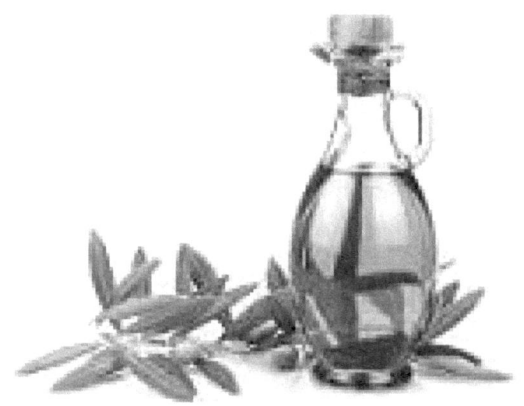

Procedure:

Step 1: Apply warm extra-virgin olive oil on the stretch marks and massage the skin to improve blood circulation.

Step 2: Allow it on the skin for half an hour before you wash it off. This is to allow the vitamins to be fully absorbed in the skin.

Alternatively you can mix Vinegar with olive oil and water. This mixture is used as a night cream to keep the skin moisturized. Using this method, you won't need to apply extra-virgin olive oil during the day.

WATER

The importance of water in getting rid of stretch marks is significant. Water aids in detoxification and restores the elasticity of the skin.

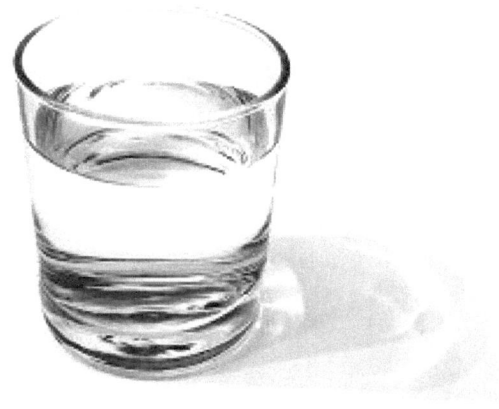

Drink at least 2 glasses of water at once, and ten times throughout the day. Involve in activities that will help your body to crave water, such as exercising.

Also, you can opt for flavored drinks in order to improve fluid intake.

Your aim is to keep your body hydrated by drinking at least 10 glasses of water daily.

In this case you are to avoid soda or coffee as much as possible.

Exercise

Exercising is one of the best methods of getting rid of stretch marks caused by weight gain.

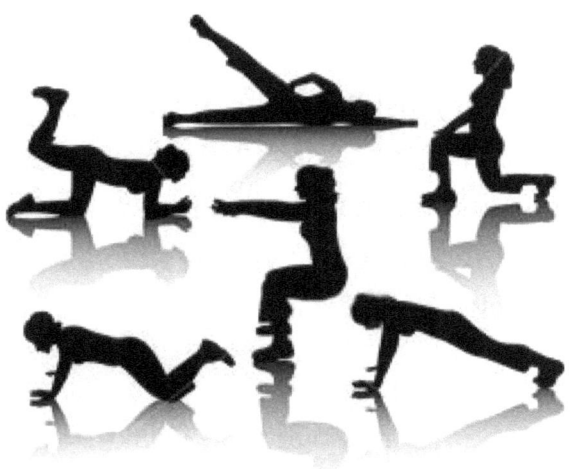

Exercises such as swimming, abdominal crunches and sit-ups help very much in toning the muscles, therefore helps in the process of healing the stretch marks.

Stretch Marks on Buttocks and Hips

Exercise procedure:

Step 1: Lie on your back flat, with your knees touching each other.

Step 2: Lift the left leg to create a 90% angle.

Step 3: Do the same for the other leg until you get tired.

Alternatively, you can lay face down, with your arms on the side. Lift one leg up and down, then the other.

Practice this exercise daily in order to get positive results.

CHAPTER FIVE: Myths and Facts about Stretch Marks

Myth 1: Stretch marks disappear with weight loss.

Myth Debunked:

Contrary to the belief that weight loss can make stretch mark disappear, weight loss is among the common and regular causes of stretch marks. When weight loss becomes drastic, especially in people who are obese, it may result to severe case of stretch mark.

The best way to prevent this kind of development is by involving in gradual weight loss through exercises and diet adjustment. The physical activity the body is exposed to during a progressive weight loss affects the skin elasticity, determining whether the skin is going to be prone to stretch marks or not.

Myth 2: Cannot be prevented

Myth Debunked:

The only people that may not be able to avoid stretch marks are those with family history. Even the hereditary factor can be controlled to reduce the development of stretch marks.

One way to prevent the occurrence is by drinking more water. Staying hydrated keeps the skin naturally moisturized, especially during pregnancy.

Home remedies such as pure Shea butter, virgin coconut oil and cocoa butter are recommended; to be used on the skin to reduce the possibility of developing stretch marks.

Also in preventing the occurrence, regular exercise and the consumption of protein rich foods is very important to have the skin elastic and to withstand stretches and strains

When extreme weight loss or gain is expected due to dieting or pregnancy, performing regular workout will keep the skin healthy.

In a recent study, it was found that regular massage helps in preventing stretch marks, although the massages must be regular and must be concentrated on places prone to stretch marks like the belly, hip, thighs, arm etc.

Myth 3: They are caused only by skin stretching.

Myth Debunked:

We all know that weight loss and gain bring about stretch marks, as a result of stretching of the skin. Also pregnant women develop stretch marks as a result of the same stretching of the skin. But genes do play a significant role in determining when they will appear and how chronic the stretch marks are.

This means that if your sister or mother have them you are likely to have some.

Other factors that determine the occurrence of stretch marks include hormonal changes, amount of body fat and skin type.

Myth 4: Treatments are covered by insurance.

Myth Debunked:

Stretch mark treatment is mostly classified by insurance agencies as cosmetic procedures as it involves the same dermatological procedures, so they are not covered. Although, it would be important to ask your health insurance provider for clarification on specific stretch mark treatment methods.

Once you are able to familiarize with the use of home remedies for your skin care, you may not need clinical procedures to get rid of stretch marks, regardless how bad they are.

Myth 5: Medicinal drugs do not cause stretch marts.

Myth Debunked:

Taking medicinal drugs regularly can cause stretch marks. Such drugs include steroids and pills; this is because when used incorrectly they might lead to increased weight gain. The uncontrolled weight gain therefore stretches the skin, making the lines to appear.

There are alternative ways you can reduce the risk of developing stretch marks while you use medicinal drugs. Ask your physician for options.

Myth 6: Stretch marks can be treated.

Myth Debunked:

It is an actual skin trauma that begins on the second layer of the skin, the dermis. Dermatological procedures can help in improving the appearance of the skin, but the best way to be free from stretch marks is by involving in regular activities like the use of essential oil and other natural procedures.

All being said, stretch marks can only go away gradually.

The procedures help in the increase of the production of collagen, bringing about soft skin and also minimize discoloration. The natural methods also aid in the replacement of damaged skins.

In many cases, dermatological procedures offered by most physicians are aimed at tightening the skin, which include the use of skin products that usually don't work for post-treatment application.

The best way to improve the skin is by intensifying your workout sessions; drinking more liquid and improving your diet.

Myth 7: Diet does not prevent stretch marks.

Myth debunked:

Apart from the effect of the food you eat on the amount of weight you gain daily, it has been proven that certain types of food help in improving the skin. Healthy balanced diet helps your system, the whole physiological and psychological well-being, including the skin is actively related to the kind of food you eat.

Myth 8: Stretch marks mainly affect women.

Myth debunked:

Obviously women are more susceptible to stretch mark due to the regular changes their bodies go through, but men also get affected by stretch marks. Body builders and athletes are more prone to stretch marks due to excessive stretching of the skin. Men are also anxious of stretch marks and as well as women, want to lose them.

Apparently, the occurrence of stretch marks among men is less often than women. This is because women store more fat in their bodies than men. Unlike women, men tend to have more muscles and less fat.

Myth 9: Stretch marks only occur in stomach

Myth debunked:

Since stretch marks occur mostly among women due to pregnancy, it is easier to conclude that it only occur in the stomach. But stretch marks can also be noticed around the upper arm, knee creases, thighs, buttocks, calves, elbow creases, lower back and the breasts.

In women, stretch marks are common around the stomach and the lower back while in men, they occur mostly around the elbow and knee creases.

Myth 10: Skinny people cannot get stretch marks

Myth debunked:

Stretch marks also occur in skinny people due to genetic and hormonal factors. Hormonal changes which are common among teens and preteens may bring about the occurrence of stretch marks. And these changes occur regardless of weight, age or gender.

In rare cases, health issues such as Cushing's syndrome and Marfan syndrome cause the problem. Also, the prolonged use of topical corticosteroids can also be associated with rapid development of stretch marks.

Myth 11: Tanning removes stretch marks

Myth debunked:

Yes, tanning has a concealing effect that covers the stretch marks, but in some cases tanning can make stretch marks bold, since they are scar tissues.

Tanning darkens the skin but leaves scar tissues even bolder. So the mature silvery colored stretch marks may become bolder with tanning.